Clinical Practice Guidelines for Complex-ADHD

Craig B. Liden, MD

ISBN: 9798646873898

Acknowledgments

The Clinical Guidelines for Complex-ADHD project has been a team effort. Many members of the BWC have contributed to its creation. I want to acknowledge and express my gratitude to all of my teammates who have brought this book to life. In particular, I want to thank the following individuals:

- Beth Hendrickson: Director of Marketing, Senior Editor
- Jane Reck: Director of Clinical Services, Associate Editor
- Terri West: Associate Medical Director
- Sharon Spiaggi: Intake/Patient Care Coordinator
- Zack Wessel: Director of Clinical Testing
- Sam Caurdy and Jennifer Naciri: Behavioral Health Coordinators
- MaryJo Kondrit, Jill Todd, Amy Elliott, Erica Brown and all those professionals who have played a role in our clinical program over the past 40 years.
- Sherri Terravecchia: Office Coordinator and Shelby Eckenrod: Office Assistant
- Our patients and participants in my workshops over many years whose critical feedback has helped me continuously refine and improve my approach.

Disclaimers and Disclosures

CONTENTS

Reflections from a Silver-Haired Physician

In 1995, I was accepted to make a presentation to the First International Conference on Research and Practice in Attention Deficit Disorder in Jerusalem, Israel. The title of my talk was "TRANSACT: Toward A Standard of Care for ADD." I described the unique transdisciplinary system I had created for assessing, diagnosing, and managing ADD and associated co-existing conditions, and I presented data that demonstrated the efficacy of my system in addressing the needs of children and adults with ADD along with its cost effectiveness and efficiency.

At the same conference, Dr. Russell Barkley, a renowned research psychologist and expert on ADD, gave the keynote address during which he discussed the role of Executive Functions and Self-Regulation in ADD. This was a seminal talk that expanded our horizons about what ADD really is.

My talk in Jerusalem did not create as big a splash as Barkley's, but it was very well received and helped establish the legitimacy of my program in the eyes of some of my peers and health care administrators interested in replicating my model and, most importantly, with adults with ADD and parents of children with ADD. It opened the door for me to travel across the country and educate thousands of individuals about ADD, its consequences, and the answers that my system provides. It motivated me to write several practical books translating and applying my approach and the learning I have gained in applying my model with more than 10,000 individuals over more than 40 years.

Interestingly, 25 years later Barkley and I, traveling very different paths, wound up at the same destination. My clinical experience has taught me that ADD is at the core of many of the most significant health, educational, and social problems facing society. Barkley's longitudinal research has demonstrated that ADD, if undiagnosed or inadequately treated, can lead to significant co-morbidities and almost a 13-year reduction in lifespan.[1] A leading professional society concerned with ADD consummated the serious nature of ADD by coining the new term **Complex-ADHD** to describe it. They have issued new clinical guidelines[2] that are summarized in this book.

Yet, despite these profound realizations about a problem (ADHD) that might affect as much as 15% of our population, society and key players in it, have not really latched onto these findings and initiated efforts to address them. In fact, quite the opposite seems to be happening:

- Why aren't we screening at-risk populations like obese individuals who have a 25-40% risk of having ADD? Or teenage drivers who, if they have ADD, have a 6-8 fold higher incidence of traffic accidents? Or entering college freshmen whose possible ADD could reduce their chances of graduating to only 20%.

- Why aren't physicians including an evaluation for possible ADD in their work-up with patients who have chronic constipation and other bowel problems to which we know it can be a major contributor? Or in patients with mental health problems like anxiety and depression who aren't responding to typical treatments that generally work, when we know that untreated ADD can lead to chronic anxiety and recurrent failure resulting in chronic depression?

- Why do pharmacists question the dosages and all-day regimens of stimulants prescribed by experts as determined after thorough evaluation and trial testing while passively filling prescriptions by non-specialists for school day-only administration when we know ADD is an all-day, all-life problem?

- Why would a health insurance company refuse to reimburse prescriptions written by ADD experts with years of experience because their statistical reviews find them to be "outliers" as opposed to questioning whether the "other" prescribers are doing thorough evaluations before diagnosing and treating ADD and prescribing sub-therapeutic treatments that can increase patient morbidity and mortality? Who are the *real* outliers?

After years of reflection, I have come to the realization that leaders in the field like me and Dr. Barkley and professional organizations like the Society for Developmental and Behavioral Pediatrics and the American Academy of Pediatrics haven't done a good enough job increasing public and professional awareness about **Complex-ADHD** and its impact and have fallen short in advocating for proper, high quality care for **Complex-ADHD**.

This book is my attempt to kick off a movement! By translating the recommendations of the SDBP and AAP into simpler terms and providing an example, my Being Well Center, of how to successfully implement and sustain quality care for ADD, I hope this book will be a catalyst for change by professionals, insurers, governmental agencies, along with individuals living with or touched by ADD. Let our simple mantra be:

DON'T LET ADD SUBTRACT FROM LIFE!

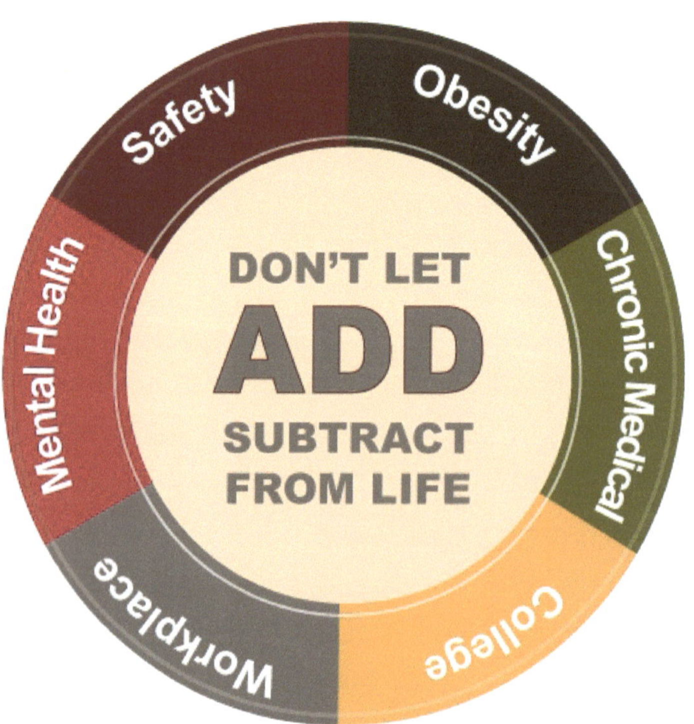

OVERVIEW of Clinical Practice Guidelines

We now know that ADD/ADHD is a serious problem that if left undiagnosed or inadequately treated can adversely affect all domains of an individual's life and lead to more than a 12-year reduction in life span.[1] It is a key contributor to many of the most challenging health, educational, and social problems we face as a society. Professional societies have recognized this fact by coining the term **"Complex-ADHD"** and updating their guidelines[2] for optimal care of this daunting problem.

This book is intended to provide an overview of these guidelines and present a model program, The Being Well Center, that has successfully implemented them over four decades with more than 10,000 patients. Specifically, it is intended to do the following:

- Help clinicians define what their appropriate role should be in assessing, diagnosing, and treating **Complex-ADHD.**
- Assist professionals (physicians, educators, mental health professionals, pharmacists, etc.), who are either

establishing programs or evaluating the quality of care provided to patients with **Complex-ADHD** in existing programs.

- Guide insurers and governmental agencies in setting policies and procedures regarding reimbursement of care and pharmaceutical formularies needed to optimally treat **Complex-ADHD** and reduce long-term morbidity and mortality.
- Serve as a resource for patients and significant others to self-advocate for high quality of care for **Complex-ADHD**.

The following check-list, based upon the opinion/research of experts in the ADHD field, serves as a synopsis of the key take-aways:

<table>
<tr><td colspan="2">Clinical Practice Guidelines for Complex ADHD
Check the box that best answers each question:</td><td>YES</td><td>NO</td></tr>
<tr><td>1.</td><td>Does the clinician directing the care have advanced training in ADHD?</td><td></td><td></td></tr>
<tr><td>2.</td><td>Does the clinician have several years of hands-on experience working with a significant number of Complex-ADHD patients across the life span?</td><td></td><td></td></tr>
<tr><td>3.</td><td>Does the clinician have ready access to a multidisciplinary team of professionals in related disciplines to consult with and assist in providing care?</td><td></td><td></td></tr>
<tr><td>4.</td><td>Does the clinician/program conduct a comprehensive evaluation gathering data from multiple sources (interviews, questionnaires, reports, etc.) about the whole person before making the diagnosis of Complex-ADHD?</td><td></td><td></td></tr>
<tr><td>5.</td><td>Does the program conduct some form of hands-on assessment of the individual's attention and executive functioning along with other relevant skills and abilities?</td><td></td><td></td></tr>
<tr><td>6.</td><td>Does the clinician/program obtain a medical history and conduct a physical and mental status examination?</td><td></td><td></td></tr>
<tr><td>7.</td><td>Does the clinician/program make the diagnosis of Complex-ADHD based upon established criteria (e.g., DSM)?</td><td></td><td></td></tr>
<tr><td>8.</td><td>Does the clinician/program provide multimodal treatment plans that include supportive counseling, medication, and other therapies as indicated?</td><td></td><td></td></tr>
<tr><td>9.</td><td>Does the clinician/program identify co-morbid/co-existing conditions and provide treatment for them or make referrals to others with necessary expertise?</td><td></td><td></td></tr>
<tr><td>10.</td><td>Does the clinician conduct some form of systematic, objective trial testing when medication is indicated?</td><td></td><td></td></tr>
<tr><td>11.</td><td>Does the clinician provide medication regimens based upon systematic procedures that provide the patient with symptom resolution throughout the waking day?</td><td></td><td></td></tr>
<tr><td>12.</td><td>Does the clinician conduct regular monitoring of medication efficacy, compliance, and side effects?</td><td></td><td></td></tr>
<tr><td>13.</td><td>Does the clinician/program have familiarity with the long-term consequences of Complex-ADHD across the lifespan and provide anticipatory guidance to avoid future problems?</td><td></td><td></td></tr>
<tr><td>14.</td><td>Does the clinician/program include significant others in the evaluation and treatment process?</td><td></td><td></td></tr>
</table>

Figure 1: Clinical Practice Guidelines

A "NO" response to *any* of these questions should raise a red flag for:

- Individual clinicians who should consider referring the patient with **Complex-ADHD** to someone with greater experience and expertise
- Program directors who should consider expanding or refining their program
- Outside reviewers who should realize that the program they are evaluating falls short of the current standard of care for **Complex-ADHD**
- Payers who should be aware that their policies and procedures may be resulting in substandard care which could increase the morbidity and mortality of **Complex-ADHD**
- Patients/significant others who should look elsewhere for quality care for **Complex-ADHD**

INTRODUCTION

The Standard of Care for ADD/ADHD

The Being Well Center: An Outlier Excelling in the Diagnosis, Assessment, and Treatment of Complex-ADHD

In late 2018, Barkley, a pioneer in the ADHD field, published updated results from his long-term longitudinal study of a cohort of individuals with ADHD which demonstrated that undiagnosed/inadequately treated ADHD results in nearly a 13-year reduction in lifespan.[1] This dramatic finding spurred the Society for Developmental and Behavioral Pediatrics (SDBP) to re-examine their position regarding ADHD and coin the term **Complex-ADHD** to describe individuals who present with symptoms of ADHD before the age of 4 years or after age 12 years or experience one or more co-morbidities in addition to their ADHD symptoms.[2] They advocate that individuals with **Complex- ADHD** require greater professional expertise or experience beyond the typical family physician or pediatrician to be properly assessed, diagnosed and treated.

Previously, in 2019 the American Academy of Pediatrics presented revised guidelines for ADHD and identified barriers to achieving their new mandates including: inadequate clinician training regarding ADHD, limitations on number of visits and inadequate reimbursement for ADHD services by payers, restrictive formularies, quantity limits, and medication approval processes, and challenges in the organization and staffing of clinical practices.[3] These barriers have led to inefficient and ineffective care models that do not comprehensively address the needs of patients with **Complex-ADHD.**

In the face of these challenges, The Being Well Center (BWC) has stood out for many years as a clinical program that has overcome these barriers by using innovative multidisciplinary staffing along with highly structured, comprehensive diagnostic and treatment protocols to successfully address the needs of the patient with **Complex- ADHD.**

The BWC's comprehensive assessments lead to accurate diagnoses and comprehensive multimodal treatment plans that include individualized counseling targeted to the patient's unique needs and systematic medication trial testing to define safe all-day treatment regimens that address the impact of ADHD throughout the day in all life spheres. Monitoring of The BWC's **Complex-ADHD** patients reveals greater than an 80% success rate and a 94% patient satisfaction rate.

The BWC is a model that needs to be embraced and replicated in order for society to successfully address the massive public health problem **Complex-ADHD** represents.

CHAPTER 1: Clinical Practice Guidelines

In February 2020, The Society of Developmental and Behavioral Pediatrics (SDBP) coined the term **"Complex-ADHD"** [2] to describe individuals with ADHD who have one or more co-existing condition(s) or other factor(s) that complicates the evaluation and treatment of their ADHD:

- Presenting at an early (<4 years) or late (>12 years) age
- Having a co-existing/co-morbid condition (medical, psychiatric, or developmental)
- Moderate to severe impact of symptoms on daily functioning in any life sphere
- Primary care physician being uncertain about the diagnosis
- Inadequate response to previous treatment

The SDBP strongly recommends that children and adolescents with suspected or diagnosed **Complex-ADHD** should be referred by their primary care provider to a clinician with specialized training or expertise in ADHD for a comprehensive assessment, diagnosis, and implementation of a multimodal treatment plan.

It states that the assessment should employ an evidence-based, developmentally appropriate, culturally sensitive approach which includes data from multiple settings and sources (home, school, community) to verify any previous diagnoses and assess for co-existing conditions. It should include a comprehensive medical history and physical and psychological assessments based upon presenting problems, their severity, the degree of functional impairments, the individual's cognitive/developmental level, and the treating clinician's judgment.

The assessment should lead to the development and initiation of an individualized inter-professional, multimodal treatment plan that includes psycho-education about ADHD and evidence-based behavioral and educational interventions addressing the key functional domains that are associated with long-term outcome.

Treatment of **Complex-ADHD** should address any identified co-existing conditions coupled with developmentally appropriate strategies for self-management, skill building, and prevention of adverse outcomes. The guidelines state that it is often necessary to combine these approaches with pharmacological treatments often utilizing more than one agent with stimulant medications considered to be first-line treatment. Pharmacological monitoring of the following domains should occur at least 2 to 4 times per year:

- ADHD symptoms and functioning
- Symptoms, impairments, and functioning related to co-existing conditions
- Physical parameters: weight and height/cardiovascular markers (BP/HR)

- Psychosocial stressors
- Identification and promotion of strengths
- Side effects from treatments

Given that ADHD is a chronic condition that often persists into adulthood, the SDBP recommends that the treatment of **Complex-ADHD** should include ongoing monitoring of patients throughout the life span with particular emphasis on key developmental transition points (e.g., primary to secondary school, starting college, starting career, getting married, having children, etc).

CHAPTER 2: The Rational Behind the Guidelines

Over the past decade there has been increasing awareness and acceptance that ADHD is much more than the prototypical 7-year-old hyperactive, impulsive boy who can't sit still to learn and whose behavior is a handful to manage. We now know that ADHD is a genetically-based collection of attentional weaknesses and executive dysfunctions that most affected individuals don't grow out of. When left undiagnosed and inadequately treated, ADHD is at the core of many of our most serious health and societal problems. [See Figure 2]

The seriousness of ADHD was driven home by Russell Barkley in late 2018 when he published the results of his long-term follow-up study of the Hyperactive Child Syndrome which demonstrated a 12.7 year reduction in life span[1] if undiagnosed/improperly treated ADHD persists into adulthood! This certainly served as a wake-up call for leaders in the field (e.g., SDBP) to step up and advocate for significant refinements and improvements of how we assess and treat **Complex-ADHD.**[2]

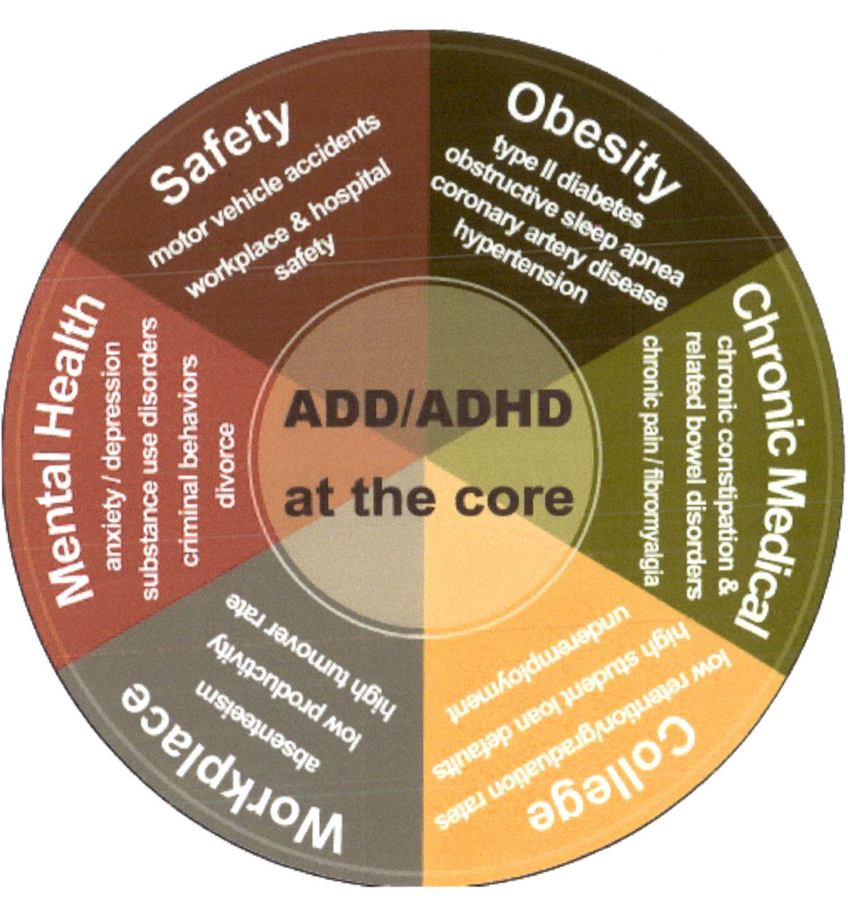

Figure 2: ADD/ADHD at the Core

CHAPTER 3: Barriers to Addressing the Mandate of Providing Excellent Care for Complex-ADHD

In October 2019, the American Academy of Pediatrics published a revision[3] to its 2011 guidelines on evaluating, diagnosing, and treating ADHD, the most common childhood neurobehavioral disorder and the second most commonly diagnosed childhood condition after asthma. National surveys have found that 9.4% of 2 to 17 year olds have been diagnosed with ADHD and community-based samples suggest a prevalence between 9 and 15%. 67% of children with ADHD have at least one co-morbidity and 18% have 3 or more co-morbidities which increase the complexity of diagnosis and treatment processes (i.e., the SDBP **Complex-ADHD** distinction).

The majority of care for children and adolescents with ADHD is provided by the child's primary care physician, particularly when it appears to be uncomplicated. Because of the high prevalence of ADHD, it is essential that primary care physicians be able to diagnose, treat, and coordinate care for ADHD or identify an appropriately experienced or expert clinician who can do so. Despite having a higher prevalence than most other conditions dealt with by primary care physicians, ADHD is often seen as being different from other conditions and beyond the purview of primary care. This can result in minimization of the patient's symptoms and parental concerns, delay in diagnosis and worsening of the child's functional ability in multiple life spheres, or the provision of sub-therapeutic interventions behaviorally, educationally, and pharmacologically that are often poorly complied with due to lack of efficacy.

In issuing their updated guidelines, the AAP also identified other barriers to the provision of timely diagnosis and treatment for children and adolescents with ADHD[4]:

1. Limited access to quality care because of inadequate training of pediatricians and other primary care providers in developmental-behavioral and mental health arenas during their residencies and other post-doctoral training. This is compounded by a national shortage of child and adolescent psychiatrists and developmental-behavioral pediatricians.

2. Inadequate payment by third party payers for needed services and payment mechanisms that impede the delivery of quality, comprehensive care for ADHD. Many payers have restrictive service and/or medication approval processes which prevent patients from receiving or continuing needed care and treatment. Limitation of medication options, mandatory step therapy, frequent formulary changes

resulting in patient destabilization and disproportionately high copays for mental health care and psychotropic medications are additional obstacles to quality care.

3. Furthermore, payments for mental health and other cognitive services are frequently lower than paid for physical health care services. This becomes problematic for patients and clinicians dealing with **Complex-ADHD** which often requires more frequent and longer visits to satisfactorily address the complicated issues involved. The administration of recommended assessment tools, like rating scales, are often not reimbursed. Time consuming coordination of care activities including communication with parents, teachers, and other interested parties is uncompensated. A recent AAP survey found that 41% of members cited inadequate reimbursement as the reason they don't provide mental health counseling and 46% said they would add a mental health professional to their staff if reimbursement could be guaranteed.

4. Payers' processes regarding medication approval create major challenges for optimally treating **Complex-ADHD**. Despite best practice evidence-based guidelines, insurance companies often favor one medication over others. Cost seems to be a key determinant. Physician appeals of medication denials are often reviewed by "peers" who have limited

knowledge about **Complex-ADHD** and lack pediatric experience and familiarity with the effect of the patient's co-morbid conditions or developmental stage. Step therapy protocols at treatment initiation require time consuming treatment failures before an effective therapeutic regimen is determined. Formulary changes may force medication adjustments on a patient who is well-controlled leading to increased morbidity and the emergence of new side effects. In addition, the assumption that generic psychotropic medications are equivalent in efficacy and duration to brand-name is not always accurate. When a patient switches insurance plans, formularies frequently change and clinicians have to spend extensive time advocating for the patient's current regimen or developing a new one that results in added cost and stress for everyone.

5. Challenges in Practice Organization. Quality comprehensive care for **Complex-ADHD** requires additional clinician time for complex visits, consultations, and communication with other care team members and staff time to coordinate delivery of chronic care. This entails creating a practice environment that is patient and family centered and that promotes the development of a strong working relationship that encourages active patient/family participation in their care. This may entail modifying office systems. Electronic systems (EHR), which can be expensive, can help address some of these barriers

and enhance communication between various stakeholders involved who can't always be available at the same time. EHR systems can also facilitate data collection regarding diagnoses, symptoms, response to medications, and side effects. Telemedicine holds significant promise as a cost effective/efficient way to assess ADHD individuals, provide quality-based treatments, and monitor responses and progress.

It also means identifying, developing, and maintaining a network of community resources that can support optimal patient care. Patients with **Complex-ADHD** and their families frequently require support and strong advocacy to follow through with referrals and other recommendations. Integration of mental health services within the practice can address some of these barriers but this optimally requires the development of an innovative, integrated, collaborative care model.

The Being Well Center, my innovative program in Pittsburgh, PA, that has been providing cost effective, transdisciplinary, multimodal diagnostic and treatment services for children and adults with ADHD since the mid 1980's is described in the next chapters.

CHAPTER 4: Overview of The Being Well Center

The Being Well Center (BWC) is a medically-based team of professionals that specializes in the diagnosis and treatment of Attention Deficit Disorder (ADHD) and related co-morbidities utilizing my Being Well System. I conceptualized the underlying philosophy, TRANSACT, in 1977 and first implemented it clinically at the Child Development Unit (CDU) of Children's Hospital of Pittsburgh, which I founded and directed until 1984.

The unique features of this innovative Being Well System include an underlying philosophy, TRANSACT, that embraces individual differences and celebrates the fact that we are each unique.

The Being Well System stresses the importance of understanding that the behavior we observe in anyone is always the end product of **transactions** among a variety of things. Some of these are located within the individual and some within the individual's environment. This means that when problems arise they can never be traced to one single reason or event. Rather, problems are the result of a poor fit between factors unique to the person and those in his environment. Therefore, the first step in solving or avoiding a problem is to consider all the things that might be contributing to a **mismatch** between the individual and expectations of the environment.

In order to do this systematically, my Being Well System has taken the letters "TRANSACT" and given them special meaning. Each stands for a possible contributor to problems a person may be experiencing:

- **T**emperament: the individual's unique *temperament* or behavioral style
- **R**eadiness: the individual's *readiness* to learn a particular behavior or skill, taking into account his unique pattern of developmental strengths and weaknesses
- **A**ttention: the individual's ability to focus and sustain *attention* and to use cognitive processes to control and monitor behavior
- **N**euromaturation: the individual's *neuromaturation* including the integrity and maturity of his nervous, sensory, and other body systems
- **S**tresses: the life *stress* events present in the individual's current or past environments
- **A**ttitudes: the *attitudes* or standards that we as parents, teachers, spouses, etc. have developed about the behavior at hand
- **C**omparisons: the *comparisons* that we and others have made among many individuals at home, at work, in school, or in the neighborhood
- **T**emperament: our individual *temperament* as parents, teachers, spouses, etc.

A comprehensive team approach should be used in working with each person's problems. Each team member should be trained to understand how the major contributors interact with one another and how to develop comprehensive treatment plans.

The professionals on The Being Well System team are trained to be "transdisciplinarians" who hold on to their special area of expertise (e.g., a medical degree or Masters degree in special education, counseling, psychology, or speech and language) while acquiring a functional understanding of the basic knowledge and skills of other disciplines by participating in a four-volume TRANSACT Training Program[5]:

I – Foundations

II – Assessment

III – Treatment

IV – Administration

Steps of the TRANSACT Approach

1. Know who the individual is by surveying his/her TRANSACT Profile

2. When a problem behavior or learning difficulty occurs, identify the expectations that are not being met

3. Determine if the expectations are realistic; if not, modify them

4. If expectations are realistic, identify all factors that are contributing to the problem: TRANSACT

5. Generate a plan to address each factor:
   - Improve those factors that are changeable
   - Work around those factors that are unchangeable
   - Accept the nature of strengths and weaknesses

6. Improving factors:
   - Medical therapies
   - Remedial activities
   - Altering other factors

7. Compensating for factors:
   - Improving self-awareness
   - Improving self-control
   - Consequences/reinforcements
   - Strategies for improved self-awareness and self-control
     - Provide feedback about behavior/performance
     - Clarify expectations/limits
     - Provide structure
     - Practice and debrief
     - Provide compensatory strategies
       - Cognitive strategies
       - Reminding strategies
       - Self-monitoring strategies
       - Problem-solving strategies

8. Acceptance
   - Education and feedback
   - Effective strategies for managing difficulties
   - Support

Figure 3: Steps of the TRANSACT Approach

The majority of patients seen at the Children's Hospital CDU had ADHD. Subsequently, I established TRANSACT Health Systems on the campus of the Forbes Regional Health Center in Monroeville, PA where the TRANSACT protocols were extended to adults with ADHD. In 2003, I moved my practice from Monroeville to Gibsonia, PA to provide easier access for patients coming from West Virginia, Ohio, Northern Pennsylvania, and Western New York. I renamed the practice The Being Well Center at that time.

Over the years, I've helped other practitioners, hospitals, and clinics establish similar programs for individuals with **Complex-ADHD** utilizing the TRANSACT approach across Pennsylvania including in DuBois, Oil City, North Hills Pittsburgh, Harrisburg, Lancaster, and Reading. I also helped establish a similar program in San Salvadore, El Salvador where all of my materials were translated into Spanish.

Over a time period of more than 40 years, my programs have diagnosed and treated more than 10,000 children, adolescents, and adults with ADHD, gaining me recognition as one of the most experienced hands-on ADHD physicians in the world. Satisfaction surveys of my patients uniformly exceed 90% in all categories.

In addition, I have published numerous articles, books, monographs, and blogs regarding ADHD including:

- *Pay Attention! Answers to the Common Questions about the Diagnosis and Treatment of Attention Deficit Disorder*
- *ADD/ADHD Basics 101: How to be a Good Consumer of Diagnostic and Treatment Services for ADD/ADHD*
- *Accommodations for Success: A Guide for Creating 504 Agreements and IEP's for Children with ADD/ADHD Using the Being Well Program*
- *Get Balance! The Guide to Living a Balanced Healthy Lifestyle*
- *Dose Up! Bring Out the Best with ADHD Medication*

I have presented testimony to Congress regarding ADHD and sat on the Board of Directors of ADDA, the national adult ADHD organization. I have been invited to lecture about ADHD to medical schools, colleges and universities, professional societies and lay audiences nationally and internationally. My special expertise centers around comprehensive evaluations of individuals suspected of having ADHD, development of multimodal treatment plans, and systematic, objective management of stimulant medications used to treat ADHD. I have been a consultant to numerous pharmaceutical companies.

CHAPTER 5: The Being Well Center's Clinical Protocol for Patients Suspected of Having Complex-ADHD

Comprehensive Multi-Disciplinary Evaluation

All patients who begin involvement at The Being Well Center participate in a **comprehensive, multidisciplinary evaluation** at the onset. The initial step in this evaluation is a **Problem Definition Visit** with the Medical Director that clarifies presenting concerns, generates a history of the patient's problem(s) over his/her life span, establishes where and how they manifest, identifies what efforts have been done to address them, and reviews his/her current functional status. This visit helps to verify the patient's commitment and makes sure that The Being Well Center is the right place to meet their needs.

Assessment Components

The next step is a formal assessment that most often includes:

- **Comprehensive developmentally-appropriate questionnaires -** These questionnaires are for the patient, parents, teachers, and significant others as indicated. They assess the individual's temperament, readiness skills, attentional status and executive functioning, and review bodily and mental symptoms, past medical, educational, and psychological history including previous testing and treatments tried, life stress events, attitudes, values, and family history.

- **Probe Interview** – Once the questionnaires are completed and returned, the patient and family meets with the Associate Medical Director to probe and clarify questionnaire responses.

- **Physical Assessment** – This includes a targeted **physical examination** with vital signs, an EKG and sensory screening as indicated and a **Mental Status Evaluation**.

- **Neurodevelopmental Testing** – This involves the use of objective tests of Neuromaturational Status, Attentional Abilities, Executive Functions, Receptive, Expressive, and Pragmatic Language Skills, and Basic Academic Skills in Reading, Math, Spelling and Written Language. The neurodevelopmental testing battery includes a proprietary electronic attention test, **FACES**™**,** which is a distinctive feature analysis task that is administered on an iPad or tablet and generates objective performance data regarding attention abilities and executive functioning along with an at-risk summary score.

Wrap-Up Visit and Case Formulation - After the formal assessment is completed, the patient/family meets with the Medical Director. This includes:

- A presentation of the testing results

- Confirmation of the ADHD diagnosis if the patient meets the expanded DSM criteria utilized by The Being Well Center

- Identification of co-morbid conditions

- Proposed treatment objectives and a plan to reach these objectives

Clinical Decision Making Protocol

The results of the evaluation and treatment recommendations are documented in an eight-page **Clinical Decision Making Protocol** in the patient's record.

Multimodal Treatment Plan

The Being Well Center employs multimodal treatment plans that include:

- **Follow-Up Counseling Sessions** with a **Transdisciplinary Case Coordinator**, weekly for 4 to 6 weeks, then at least monthly for the duration of his/her involvement with The Being Well Center. These visits are done in the office or online. The objectives of these appointments include the following as indicated by the patient's unique profile:
    - Improvement of self-awareness and acceptance of ADD/ADHD and any associated co-morbidities
    - Establishment of Healthy Daily Routines for sleep, exercise, eating, and other activities of daily living
    - Acquisition of stress management strategies including various forms of mind-centering activities
    - Development of cognitive self-control strategies to facilitate better behavioral control and task performance
    - Improvement of social/communication skills
    - Generation of social decision-making strategies
    - Reduction of co-dependency in significant others
    - Implementation of weight management strategies
    - Development of organizational strategies
    - Improvement of time/task management
    - Refinement of study skills
    - Acquisition of self-advocacy strategies
    - Development of educational or workplace accommodations
- **Consultations** with school professionals, employers or other professionals involved in the patient's care.

- **Medical Therapies** under the direction of the Medical Director/Associate Medical Director and staff including medication treatments.
- **Medication Treatments** – all patients who meet the modified DSM criteria for the diagnosis of ADHD used by BWC are considered candidates for medication treatment unless contraindications are present. Use of medication involves a number of steps:
  - **Selection of a Medication -**
    - Stimulant and non-stimulant options are presented and discussed in terms of mechanism of action, duration, benefits, and side effects. The medication recommendation is based upon the patient's unique profile and needs as determined by interview, questionnaires, and baseline attention testing.
    - Once a medication is chosen, a starting dose to begin medication trial testing is selected that is the lowest dosage that can be expected to address the patient's problem based upon years of clinical experience, guidelines proposed by various professional organizations, the contemporary medical literature, and the patient's baseline testing results during the initial assessment.[6] A small prescription is issued that allows the patient to have enough medication to participate in in-office trial testing in order to establish responsiveness to the specific medication selected and to determine an optimal dose.

- o **Medication Trial Testing** – This involves:
  - A patient starting a stimulant medication participates in in-office testing using an objective test of attention, **FACES**™, a distinctive feature analysis task that I developed and standardized. The patient takes a single dose of medication (lowest indicated) at home before coming into the office at the time when the medication should be at its peak to undergo attention testing. Trial testing can also be done at home via online *TeleTesting*. Results of the trial are compared to baseline testing done without medication during the initial evaluation. If the testing shows persistent difficulties, the dose is increased and repeat testing is done until an optimal performance is achieved.
  - Once the optimal performance is achieved, the patient is prescribed a regimen based on the testing which will provide *all* day coverage. This may be achieved in a variety of ways, such as multiple doses of a short-acting medication, a single dose of a long-acting medication, a combination of a long-acting and short-acting medication, or by combining a stimulant medication with a non-stimulant.
  - Once a daily medication regimen has been initiated, the patient has a brief **Clinical Trial Assessment Appointment (CTA)** 4-5 days after the medication is started to

check for initial efficacy, tolerability, compliance, and logistical problems. After another week, the patient meets with the Medical Director or Associate for an **Extended CTA** for more in-depth probing of the efficacy of the initial regimen and to make any necessary refinements in the dosage regimen.

Important Medication Considerations

When prescribing medication for patients with ADHD, my medical team and I consider two important realities:

- Manufacturers of stimulants only need to demonstrate a 25-30% reduction in core ADHD symptoms in their trials to obtain FDA approval. Dosage recommendations in the package inserts/PDR are the FDA-approved parameters that the pharmaceutical companies must adhere to when marketing their products and are not intended to direct physician prescribing patterns. Clinically, the goal of treatment for **Complex-ADHD** should be close to 100% symptom resolution throughout the waking day, 7 days/week, 365 days/year. Therefore, providing state-of-the-art all-day medication coverage for **Complex-ADHD** using objective testing rather than subjective questions (e.g., "How's it going?") or rating forms subject to observer bias very commonly results in off-label treatment regimens that exceed manufacturer's guidelines for maximum dosages and/or frequency of administration. Many insurance companies misuse the terms "FDA-approved" and "off-label" to justify restrictive quantity limits on their formularies that can interfere with the delivery of quality care to individuals with **Complex-ADHD**.[7] There are no discernible scientific justifications for maximum dosages for any ADHD medication.[8]

- When ADHD patients are not prescribed optimal medication regimens, they often fail to comply with treatment over time because of the lack of full efficacy. Studies show that only 15% of patients who start a stimulant prescribed by general pediatricians/family medicine physicians are still on it at the end of a year. At The Being Well Center, patients have greater than 85% compliance at year's end presumably because The Being Well Center's protocols ensure that patients are prescribed an appropriate dosage regimen and are provided with counseling support and close follow-up monitoring. Compliance with a long-term multimodal treatment plan that includes an optimal all-day medication regimen may be a key to prolonging the life span of patients with **Complex-ADHD.**

Quarterly Review and Planning Visits

All patients treated at The Being Well Center participate in **Quarterly Review and Planning (QRP) Visits** every three months with the Medical Director or Associates in addition to regular counseling sessions with their Case Coordinator. At the QRP, the patient's current functioning in all life spheres and the status of and compliance with treatment for other co-morbid problems is surveyed. The patient's vital signs are collected and he/she undergoes a targeted physical examination, has repeat testing of his/her attention, participates in an interview to assess his/her mental status and to probe for possible side effects. At the end of the visit, the medication is continued or adjusted as indicated and feedback is given to the patient's Case Coordinator regarding suggested refinements of counseling objectives. Other tests (labs, drug screens, etc.) and consultations are ordered on an as-indicated basis. These QRPs continue for the duration of the patient's involvement at The Being Well Center. The significant people in a patient's life are often requested to participate in these visits in order to gather their feedback and engage them in the comprehensive treatment process.

Other Medications

The Being Well Center prescribes medications to address co-morbid anxiety, depression, insomnia, and other behavioral conditions on an as needed basis.

Other Medical Therapies

The Being Well Center also has systematic protocols for addressing common medical co-morbidities associated with ADHD including chronic constipation and obesity.

Logistics and Policies

At the appropriate stages in the process, patients/parents sign the following policy documents:

- Acknowledgement of General Office Policies
- Informed Consent for Dosages of Medication that Exceed Manufacturer's Guidelines and the Need for Compliance
- Mandated Minimum Counseling Visits If Taking Medications
- Privacy Policy
- Medication Refill Policy
- Email Policy
- Informed Consent for Online *GuideU* and the *TeleTesting* Visits
- Responsibility for Scheduling Appointments

All prescriptions are sent electronically to pharmacies after the state registry is checked and compliance with mandated BWC visits is confirmed.

CHAPTER 6: Financial Policies of
The Being Well Center

After leaving the Child Development Unit where the services that my team provided were billed through The Children's Hospital of Pittsburgh, I and my clinical programs have never been participating providers with any insurance plans. It has given me and my team the freedom to provide quality comprehensive services without being constrained by insurance companies' arbitrary, uninformed policies and inadequate reimbursements. This has allowed me and my team to spend the time, conduct the frequency of visits, and use of state-of-the-art tools required to meet the multifaceted assessment and treatment needs of patients with **Complex-ADHD**. Therefore, patients coming to The Being Well Center are self-pay unless they have out-of-network coverage through their insurance plan.

The cost of The Being Well Center's individual services is generally below that of comparable programs because of its cost effective/cost efficient service model. The Being Well Center does provide free or reduced cost services to needy patients and offers Health Scholarships through its non-profit entity, TRANSHealth.

At one point, when The Being Well Center/TRANSACT helped hospitals and community health systems in Central Pennsylvania establish wholly owned programs utilizing the TRANSACT methodology, I was approached by the senior management of Capital Blue Cross (Senior Medical Director, Vice President for Provider Affairs, and the Director of Patient Relations) with a plan to give my satellite programs a special code to submit with their billings that would give Blue Cross patients 80% reimbursement for all TRANSACT services. Their intent was to preferentially drive their patients to the TRANSACT programs where they knew they would get high quality, comprehensive care and minimize or eliminate the long-term risks of ADHD, which we now know result in nearly a 13-year reduction in lifespan. They felt that this was the right thing to do for their patients and Capital Blue Cross' bottom-line. This plan was implemented for a better part of the 1990's.

Subsequently, I proposed similar agreements with other insurance companies who refused, citing: "We know consumers change insurance plans approximately every two years. Why would we want to do something like this and pay out dollars for services that our competitors will benefit from?!" Maybe because it's the right thing to do! As it turns out, these leaders at Capital Blue Cross were ahead of their time and had a foreshadowing of the impact of **Complex-ADHD!**

Bibliography

1. Barkley RA, Fischer M. "Hyperactive Child Syndrome and Extended Life Expediency at Young Adult Follow-Up: The Role of ADHD Persistence and Other Potential Predictors." <u>J Attention Disorders</u>: Pub Med, <u>https://doi.org/10/1177/1087054718816164</u>. 2018.

2. Barbaresi WJ, Campbell L, Dickroger EA, et al. "Society for Developmental and Behavioral Pediatrics Clinical Practice: Guidelines for the Assessment and Treatment of Children and Adolescents with Complex Attention Deficit/Hyperactivity Disorder." <u>J Dev Behav, Ped 41</u>:535-557. 2020.

3. Wolraich ML, Hagam JF, Allan C, et al. AAP Subcommittee on Children and Adolescents with Attention Deficit/Hyperactivity Disorder. "Clinical Practice Guideline for the Diagnosis, Evaluation, and Treatment of Attention Deficit/Hyperactivity Disorder in Children and Adolescents." <u>Pediatrics 144</u> (4) e20192528; 2019: 1-28.

4. Wolraich, et al. "Supplemental Information: Systemic Barriers to the Case of Children and Adolescents with ADHD." <u>Pediatrics 144</u> (4) e20192528; 2019: 29-43.

5. Liden, CB, Laurie TE, Zalenski JR. *The Transact Training*

Program. Volumes 1-4. Pittsburgh, PA. Transact Health Systems; 1987.

6. Liden, CB and West, TA. *Dose Up! Bring Out the Best with ADHD Medication*. Pittsburgh, PA. TRANSHealth; 2015.

7. Ching C, Erlick GD, Paulton AS. "Evaluation of Methylphenidate Safety and Maximum Dose Titration Rationale in Attention Deficit/Hyperactivity Disorder. A Meta-Analysis." JAMA Pediatr 173 (7); 2019: 630-639.

8. Meadows, WA and Hallowell, BD. "'Off-Label' Drug Use: An FDA Regulatory Term, Not a Negative Implication of Its Medical Use." International Journal of Impotence Research. 20; 2008: 135-144.

About the Author

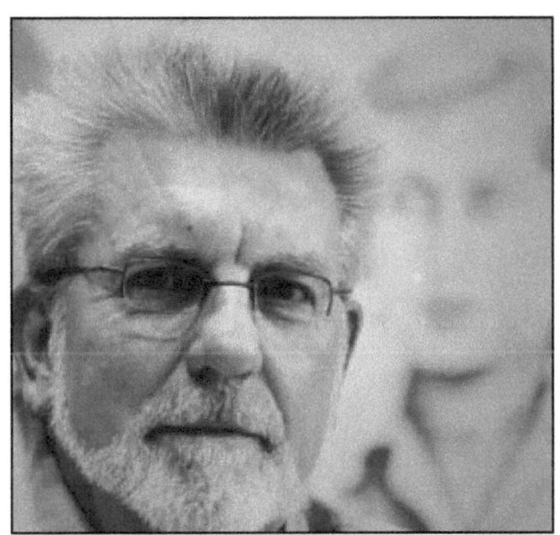

Craig B. Liden, MD
Biographical Sketch – Professional Highlights

- Attended the University of Michigan and obtained a BS cum laude
- Attended Ohio State University College of Medicine and obtained a MD with distinction
- Elected to Alpha Omega Alpha, the national medical honor society
- Completed a Pediatric Residency and a two-year postdoctoral fellowship in developmental and behavioral medicine at the Harvard University and the Children's Hospital Medical Center, Boston
- Served on the faculty at the University Of Pittsburgh School Of Medicine
- Established the Child Development Unit at the Children's Hospital of Pittsburgh

- Implemented a postdoctoral fellowship program in developmental pediatrics at the University of Pittsburgh Medical Center
- Appointed as a Center Associate at the University of Pittsburgh Learning Research and Development Center
- Created the TRANSACT Approach to developmental, learning and behavioral dysfunctions
- Founded TRANSACT health systems, Inc., served as President and Senior Medical Director, and helped establish six satellite programs across Pennsylvania
- Treated more than 10,000 patients with Attention Deficit Disorder
- Accepted to present his research to national meetings of more than 12 national organizations
- Elected to the Board of Directors of ADDA, the national Attention Deficit Disorder Association
- Provided testimony about the diagnosis and treatment of Attention Deficit Disorder to the Intergovernmental Sub-Committee of the US House of Representatives
- Invited to present a paper entitled "TRANSACT: Toward a Standard of Care for ADD" to the First International Conference of ADD in Jerusalem, Israel
- Conducted hundreds of workshops for medical, psychological and educational professionals across the US from Georgia to Alaska and internationally from Israel to El Salvador

- Written more than 30 books, chapters, and articles about Attention Deficit Disorder and other developmental/behavioral topics including: *Pay Attention! Answers to common questions about the diagnosis and treatment of Attention Deficit Disorder, Get Balance! The Guide to Living a Balanced Healthy Lifestyle, Accommodations for Success: A Guide for Creating 504 Agreements and IEP's for Children with ADD/ADHD, How to be a Good Consumer of Diagnostic/Treatment Services for ADD/ADHD,* and *Dose Up! Bring out the best with ADHD Medication*
- Served as consultant to hospitals, medical centers, universities and pharmaceutical companies regarding Attention Deficit Disorder and its diagnosis and treatment

About The Being Well Center

The Being Well Center (BWC), an internationally recognized ADD/ADHD diagnostic and treatment center, offers innovative services for the complex problems of ADD across the lifespan. Our team includes physicians, physician assistants, behavioral health coordinators, nurses, counselors, dieticians, speech pathologists, and educational experts. We provide a long-term, supportive relationship with our team of experts who listen and care. We support the carefully monitored use of medication as one part of an individualized, comprehensive, multimodal treatment plan. Over more than 40 years, we've worked with more than 10,000 people with ADD/ADHD. We know ADD!

www.thebeingwellcenter.com

About TRANShealth, Inc.

TRANShealth, Inc. is a non-profit organization that promotes the acceptance of Attention Deficit Disorder and Attention Deficit Hyperactive Disorder through education, responsible treatment, and celebration of the individual. We seek to support health care and educational programs that remove the boundaries to success at home, school, higher education and in the workplace for individuals with ADD/ADHD.

TRANShealth, Inc. is committed to playing a key role in developing more accurate, cost-effective, and efficient treatment of ADD/ADHD for the 21st century. We impact children, adults, and their families with complex health care problems and educational needs related to ADD/ADHD. We strive to increase public and professional awareness of the virtues of treating the whole person, not just the disorder of ADD/ADHD. www.addbasics.org

TRANSlations Press
4156 Kenneth Drive
Pittsburgh, PA 15044-5234

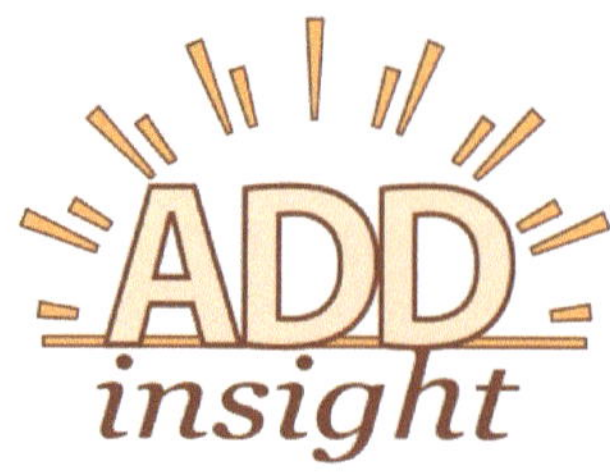

Despite affecting between 9-15% of the population, ADHD does not make it into the top 25 reasons for a doctor's visit. Yet the consequences of undiagnosed or inadequately treated ADHD riddle lists of serious causes of morbidity and mortality!

ADHD Insight is committed to increase society's awareness of **ADHD's Risk Wheel**:

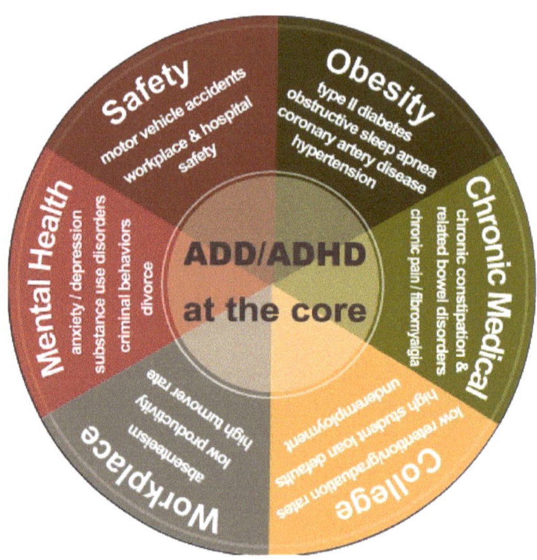

We seek to inform and advocate for what individuals with ADHD and their families, physicians, educators, employers, pharmacists, insurers, and government agencies can do to reduce the risk. Our mantra is: *Don't let ADD subtract from life!*
For More Information: **www.addinsight.org**